Healing
Is a
Journey

Blue Mountain Arts®

New and Best-Selling Titles

By Susan Polis Schutz:
To My Daughter with Love on the Important Things in Life
To My Son with Love

By Douglas Pagels:
For You, My Soul Mate
Required Reading for All Teenagers
The Next Chapter of Your Life
You Are One Amazing Lady

By Marci:
Friends Are Forever
10 Simple Things to Remember
To My Daughter
To My Mother
To My Sister
You Are My "Once in a Lifetime"

By Wally Amos, with Stu Glauberman:
The Path to Success Is Paved with Positive Thinking

By M. Butler and D. Mastromarino:
Take Time for You

By James Downton, Jr.:
Today, I Will... Words to Inspire Positive Life Changes

By Carol Wiseman:
Emerging from the Heartache of Loss

Anthologies:
A Daughter Is Life's Greatest Gift
A Son Is Life's Greatest Gift
Dream Big, Stay Positive, and Believe in Yourself
God Is Always Watching Over You
Hang In There
The Love Between a Mother and Daughter Is Forever
Nothing Fills the Heart with Joy like a Grandson
The Peace Within You
There Is Nothing Sweeter in Life Than a Granddaughter
Think Positive Thoughts Every Day
When I Say I Love You
Words Every Woman Should Remember

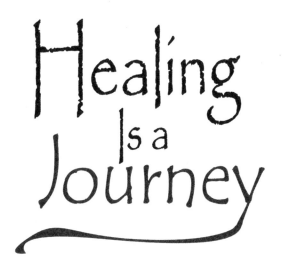

Healing Is a Journey

*Find your own path
to hope, recovery,
and wellness*

Minx Boren, MCC

Blue Mountain Press™
Boulder, Colorado

Dedication

To each of my clients, with deep appreciation for your trust in me and in the coaching process. As we have embarked together on a journey toward healing, I applaud not only your courage and determination but also acknowledge the ways I, too, have been changed in the process.

Library of Congress Catalog Card Number: 2013043684
ISBN: 978-1-59842-795-0

⋔ and Blue Mountain Press are registered in U.S. Patent and Trademark Office.
Certain trademarks are used under license.

Printed in China.
First Printing: 2014

✸ This book is printed on recycled paper.

This book is printed on paper that has been specially produced to be acid free (neutral pH) and contains no groundwood or unbleached pulp. It conforms with the requirements of the American National Standards Institute, Inc., so as to ensure that this book will last and be enjoyed by future generations.

Library of Congress Cataloging-in-Publication Data

Boren, Minx.
Healing is a journey : finding your own path to hope, recovery, and wellness / Minx Boren.
     pages cm
ISBN 978-1-59842-795-0 (trade pbk. : alk. paper) 1. Self-confidence. 2. Resilience (Personality trait) 3. Hope. I. Title.
BF575.S39B67 2014
158--dc23

2013043684

Blue Mountain Arts, Inc.
P.O. Box 4549, Boulder, Colorado 80306

Table of Contents

Introduction

In every life there will be joys and sorrows. The question becomes how to savor each of the joys and navigate our way through the sorrows that must be faced. The answer lies in our capacity to respond to all that life brings with composure, authenticity, courage, resilience, and resourcefulness.

Composure means staying calm and levelheaded in the midst of the inevitable storms that rise, swell, and then subside throughout the journey of a single life. Authenticity requires that we each find our own path, our own unique ways of being and doing what is ours to do. Yes, of course, it is helpful to learn from what others have done in challenging times, but ultimately, we must each choose our own path toward healing and wellness. Courage becomes available when we make those choices based on that which we are fervently drawn toward, value, and hold dear. Resilience and resourcefulness involve our ability to draw upon our readiness and our will and willingness to do the next best thing... and then the next.

Even in the midst of a crisis, whether of body, mind, or spirit, there is something within that guides us and gives us the strength and determination to heal in the fullest sense of the word, which is *to become whole*. Taking time and making space to know oneself—and to make choices from that awareness—is the first and best gift toward healing that we can give ourselves. Knee-jerk reactions and decisions that come from fear interfere with accessing our own truths and deep wisdom, which are at the core of finding our way to true well-being and a fulfilling life.

Since you are holding this book in your hands, my hope and intention, dear reader, is that you will use it as a guide on your own personal healing journey. With this in mind, I invite you to find your own best way to meander through this book, whether that means reading it from cover to cover or opening it to a random page when you are seeking inspiration, noticing both what is written and your own response.

However you decide to embark, I wish you good travels.

In the spirit and adventure of it all,

— Minx Boren

healing is a journey
sometimes long and slow
other times undertaken in big
determined strides
across a sometimes daunting
other times confusing landscape

and yet in truth
there is no actual destination
no momentous endpoint to be reached
where one thrusts a flag into the ground
and declares the exploration to wellness
complete

at least not as long
as one still draws breath
and navigates the sometimes quiet
other times tumultuous seas of life

and so it seems
what is ours to do on this sacred voyage
is to steer our way through
the endless swells and shallows
that rise and fall breath by breath
with courage and resilience
with joy and hope
with gratitude and faith
and a whole lot more

The Paradox of Healing

Have you ever considered that healing can be completely paradoxical? It is about doing both more *and* less. It is about hope coupled with a positive outlook, *and* it is about being totally accepting of what is quite simply so in the moment. It is about tapping into our own inner strength, wisdom, and resilience, *and* it is about asking for and accepting help. Ultimately healing requires both extraordinary selfishness (in the most self-loving sense of the word) *and* great compassion for both ourselves and others.

Doing More and Doing Less...
When a crisis arises, we want to do something... anything... everything. We research and experiment, spending time, money, and energy to explore first one approach, treatment, or strategy and then another. When the crisis is a physical one, often we find the need to try *everything*—special nutrients, appropriate exercises, healing practices such as visualization and meditation, and more. Yet our bodies have their own healing rhythm and will not be cajoled or coerced to go beyond their limitations to accommodate endless agendas and expectations. More than anything, what we need to learn is how to be gentle and patient with ourselves as, step by step, we discern our own healing journey.

Sometimes
it is all just too much
too much to fathom
too much to analyze
too much to accept
too much to do

sometimes
it is better to just let go
of all the problems
of all the tasks
of all the burdens
that weigh us down

sometimes
the greatest gift we can give ourselves is
to walk away
to walk out from under
to walk into the daylight
and to warm our souls

sometimes
when we return
our absence will have allowed for a shift
and the burdens seem
somehow easier than before

then sometimes
we must remember to be grateful
and to rest in the assuredness
that we are enough after all

Hope and Acceptance...

Hope is a survival trait. Without it, we lose heart, and without heart, we become susceptible to despair. When we can no longer see any options, we are liable to give in or give up. To keep hope alive is to hold a positive vision for the future. Yet to be fully present in our own life, we must also be willing to *be with* what is true in the moment. If we are always waiting for *when—when I am stronger, pain-free, thinner, healthier, wealthier, married, divorced, hired, retired, etc.*—before we can enjoy where we are right now or commit to something we are passionate about or dare to explore something different, then we may never experience newfound joys or reach beyond the status quo.

Self-Reliance and Receptivity...

Our response-*ability*, that is to say our ability to respond to the circumstances of our lives, is an important key to healing. Ultimately we must each decide for ourselves what is best, most curative, and most nurturing. If not, we give away our power and, with it, our will. Yet none of us is wise enough, resourceful enough, or strong enough alone. The ability to balance self-reliance with being receptive to all manner of help and support is another essential component of the healing process.

the time to remember
to love the world is
when hope seems out of reach
when the world seems
all too gray and each day
feels all too dismal and dank
when life simply refuses
to cooperate with your
best laid plans and most
cherished desires

that is the time to remember
the sound of cardinals chirp chattering
in the nearby trees
and the lizard's red throat
celebrating each breath
that is the time to remember
the way flowers turn sunward
offering their glorious colors
to just this very day
no matter whether anyone is watching

to recall life's goodness
in the easy times is... well... easy
to stay open to beauty
when everything conspires
to cloud one's view
is something else entirely

Selfishness and Compassion...
Healing is about a commitment to extraordinary
self-care that grows from a willingness to listen
deeply to our own needs, preferences, and inklings
and then invest the time and energy needed to fully
nurture ourselves. Often this requires saying "No!"
to the requests of others in order to conserve our
strength and attend to our own process. Yet our
own pain can also awaken us more fully to the pain
of another, and that awareness often inspires us to
reach out and touch someone, to say "I understand"
with deep awareness and compassion. The great
miracle is that, as we open our hearts to others,
we encourage our own healing process as well.

It is important to remember that healing includes
becoming more and more authentic and choosing to
do more of those things that bring joy into our lives.
Much is revealed to us when we pay loving attention
to who we are, what really matters to us personally,
and how we can make judicious choices that honor
our whole self.

how we heal

like a snake
shedding an outgrown skin

like a rose
slowly revealing our splendor

like an eagle
taking flight into expanding vistas

like a sunflower
turning toward the light

like a beaver
eager to build something worthwhile

like a cat
content (sometimes) to curl up and be stroked

like a tree
stretching high and wide

like an owl
attuned to the darkness and able to see beyond it

like a fish
     finding a way over, under, and around obstacles

like a waterfall
     spilling over generously

like a monk
     humbled and reverent

like a baby
     thrilled with each new sight, sound, taste, and touch

like a good banker
     carefully managing our hard-earned health

like a gypsy
     restless for new experiences

like a long gone journeyer
     grateful to be home at last

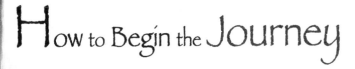

How to Begin the Journey

There are times when life is laid back and easy, when we can simply savor our moments and joyfully count the blessings that fill our days. Then there are those times when life throws a hard punch to the gut and we are—at least momentarily—down for the count, the wind and will knocked out of us. The question is this: when things get tough, how do we draw upon the strength and resilience deep within ourselves to rise to whatever occasion or challenge life has sent our way?

Whether it's a financial, physical, or emotional crisis, there is an inner resourcefulness available to each of us if we are prepared to seek it out. There are also outer resources all around us that we can tap into for support, if we are willing and wise enough to look for them.

Time and again I have learned the hard way that the answer rarely lies in simply jumping into action and getting frenetically obsessed with working harder or taking on more. We as humans are best served when we are able to first be still for a while as we step out of the frenzy of reactive "doing" long enough to listen for that intuitive inner voice. Only by taking into consideration both the whole situation and the very essence of our most authentic, sensitive, and sensible selves can we make appropriately responsive choices.

What practices awaken your resilience and fortify your strength? Perhaps it's a quiet walk in nature or just spending some time leaning against a favorite and comforting tree. Perhaps it's taking a nap or a bath or a stretch. Whatever it is, you will be well served by taking a breather and allowing the fullness of who you are and what you know to rise to the surface.

In that reflective time you can begin to assess your resources—for instance: Who are the people who support and encourage you? Where are the places that heal and recharge you? What are the possibilities, alternatives, and choices that are open or opening to you now? Whose skills and knowledge, including your own, can you tap into?

You'll know you are on the right track when you experience a sense of relief or maybe even excitement—when you begin to feel replenished rather than depleted or overwhelmed by whatever it is you decide to do.

head for your heart

When the world
is in a swirl
head for your heart

when endless confusion
clouds your horizon
and vortices of impossibilities
mar your view
head for your heart

when nothing
seems to be enough
yet wherever you turn
it all seems too much
head for your heart

when negativities
fill the air and choke off
even the merest glimmer
of breath-giving
and hope-illumined vistas

then you grasp in your
heart of hearts
that it is time
to settle down and settle in
let the grace of silence begin
to connect you to the steadfast beat
of your own true knowing

a treasure chest within
overflowing with tokens of love
and kindness
gathered along the way
a heart made strong and confident
through navigating the twists
and turns of your journey
to this moment
in time

so settle in and settle down
let your heartfullness
be your guiding star
through the bleak wilderness
of today as you open
in sweet surrender to
all your tomorrows

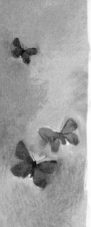

Self-Discovery Through Journaling

Perhaps you have tried to journal in the past or at least thought about it. Now is the perfect time to explore this wonderful tool for self-discovery. Journaling is a way of paying attention, of being present to what is really happening beneath the surface in your life, and of keeping a finger on the pulse of your daily moods, motivators, feelings, and expectations.

Keep in mind that your journal can become your safe place to tell your story and pour out your thoughts. Each time you put pen to paper and write about your experiences, the lessons learned, and the prospects you see emerging from the challenges of illness or pain or loss or grief, you simultaneously create an opportunity to envision your new story. The magic that can result from the practice of journaling is that you can both discover and re-create yourself on the page.

To begin, you've got to empty what's full in order to make room for something new. You cannot replenish yourself when you are bursting at your emotional seams. This is the perfect time for doing some deep soul-searching in order to uncover hidden fears, beliefs, and resentments that may no longer serve you. Next, you need to listen closely to your inner self—to all that mindful and mindless chatter—so you can really hear what's going on and eventually change what you want to say, how you want to say it, and how you want to choose to be as a result of your self-discoveries.

The effectiveness of your journaling will depend above all on five things: (1) your intention to be completely honest with yourself; (2) your commitment to write for at least ten minutes every day; (3) your openness to allow yourself to be surprised by what shows up on the page and not just write about what you've already done or already know or believe to be so; (4) your decision to not be a tough critic, to not hold on to unreasonable standards and expectations concerning both your ability to write and the worthiness or validity of what you have to say; and (5) your promise to never end your writing time on a downbeat or depressing note. No matter what you need to put down, face honestly, or let go of, always spend a few minutes at the end naming at least one thing you can do to release any negativity and one positive action you can take in pursuit of the life you want to create for yourself.

As for the best times to write—they are first thing in the morning, last thing before going to bed, and anytime an inspiration or concern moves you to seek clarity or to explore further.

Here are some journal prompts to get you started:

1. What am I feeling right now?

2. What do I need to let go of right now?

3. What can I do right now to take a step forward in my healing process?

4. What are twenty-five things I like and appreciate about myself? (If you find this difficult to do, try to be gentle and generous with yourself. You can also ask friends to tell you what they like and appreciate about you to get you started.)

5. For what and/or for whom am I grateful today?

6. What can I look forward to?

7. What is a favorite story or experience from my life that I most cherish? How can the richness of that story sustain me through the difficult times?

8. How do I want to show up during my healing journey? How do I want to be seen and known?

9. What does "healing" mean to me? In what ways can I measure and honor the healing process?

10. Is there a difference between "healing" and "wholeness"? What are the ways I can appreciate each as I move through this challenging time?

Stay awhile
here in the quiet
emptiness of a new day
do not rush too soon
to enter its impending fullness

yesterday has been
laid to rest in the folds of sleep
and today's choices and
challenges have not
yet crept over the horizon

here is when NOW is most present
just this here-now moment
when the soul returns from dreamtime
still touched by the mysteries
of other worlds and places

listen, listen
in this holy spaciousness
there is much to be savored
and more to be discovered
as today's promises emerge
out of the deep fog of sleep

and so be here now
pen in hand now
waiting for whatever
wisdom wants to find its way
onto the welcoming page

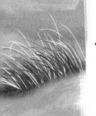

The Importance of
REALationships
in the Healing Process

The special REALationships in our lives are what light up our days and comfort us during dark nights and difficult times. It is a great blessing to be held in the loving embrace of those who have been there for us through the ups and downs of our lives. These are the people who offer their understanding and wisdom, a place at their tables, the shirts off their backs, handshakes or hugs, lists of instructions or letters of recommendation, valid praise or valuable, constructive advice, and everything else in between.

None of us is wise enough alone. The important people in our lives are the best mirrors; in their loving eyes, we can see ourselves more clearly reflected. They hold a welcoming space for the whole of us—our great gifts and strengths as well as our foolishness and foibles. They are compassionate toward our fears and past failings, but their focus remains steadfast on reminding us of our possibilities. Their presence in our lives makes all the difference. Whether family members or dear friends, what makes these relationships special are the respect and intimacy born of shared experiences and shared values. It is in the good company of these loved ones that we can show up whole and real without the need for either pretense or posturing. We do not have to guard our words or measure up to some elusive standard.

Henry David Thoreau speaks of friends as those who "cherish each other's hopes. They are kind to each other's dreams." There is no sweeter offering in all the world than that. True friendship is the ultimate treasure with which we gift ourselves simply by making time and opening heartfully to another. For all these reasons, it can also be a potent healing balm.

I have a string of prayer beads. Each bead is different and unique, and each one represents someone special in my life. There are times when I like to sit quietly and just run the beads through my fingers one by one as a way to bless and give thanks for each precious person who has walked with me at some point on my life journey.

In the end, perhaps love and its ability to quiet our minds and ease our pain is the greatest healing power of all, one that only increases as we allow our relationships to blossom all around us and spread out into larger and larger communities of caring.

*Y*our kindness arrived
at just the perfect moment
and it caught me by sweet surprise
just before I could have tumbled
into an abyss I had not seen
spreading all around me

your concern came calling
beckoning me back from the edge of my sadness
and like an offering of fragrant tea
satisfied my thirsty need
for something that could soothe
my weary and worried heart

your loving presence showed up
and offered a magical balm of comfort and caring
that spread across my whole self
in the wake of your tender reaching out
soothing the uncertainty and doubt
that had occupied all too much
of my narrowed attention

and there at the center
of your enveloping love
as your warmth melted away my frozen fears
and your voice quieted my bluesy bouts
of despondence
was the unimagined blessing of peace
and hope and on their wings
the strength to carry on

Deep Connection

We as humans are relational by nature and thrive in connection. As a species, we could not have survived otherwise because alone and on our own we were no match for mammoths or much else that threatened our very existence in prehistoric times. So we banded together, first for safety and eventually for comfort, camaraderie, and all that could develop in and through community.

The whole idea of healing circles probably also extends way back in time. Even though our lives have changed dramatically over several thousand years of existence, in times of crisis, we still gather together to tend to and befriend one another. These opportunities for deep connection and sharing, for offering sustenance and support and a whole lot more are at the very core of what it means to be fully human.

And let's not forget that actual physical touch matters as well. Studies show that orphaned infants who are kept in cribs and rarely touched or held fail to thrive. Nurses today are incorporating practices that focus on the healing powers of touch during the recovery process. Loving touch affects us not only physically but emotionally as well. We would do well to never underestimate the profound effect of being touched as well as reaching out and touching someone else.

*W*hen the world seems all too large
and you feel oh so small and inconsequential
perhaps that's the time to make time
and remember one by one
the quiet ways you have touched lives
someone near and dear perhaps
or maybe even a stranger who
was touched by your smile or
by a gentle gesture or maybe
even a small creature whose life
was spared because you swerved
out of the way thanks to your
good instincts and good heart

when the world seems all too much
and you feel all too small and of no account
that's the perfect opportunity to count
your blessings one by one
the precious ways your life has been touched
searching through your cherished
memories for all the times and ways
you were gifted with sunshine on your shoulders
or a friend perhaps who reached out a hand
or maybe even a stranger who stopped your fall
or perhaps a furry friend who nuzzled your palm
or curled up in your lap to be held
and you oh so willingly accepted these kindnesses
allowing goodness and love
to soothe your aching spirit

Step by Wobbly Step

Do you consider yourself resilient? How effectively do you manage the whole muddled messiness of being human? I admire resilience. Actually, it blows me away. There is something about being human and yet rising above human predicaments to create and achieve something beyond our wildest imaginings and in the face of incalculable obstacles. My heroes and heroines are those who make of their lives something significant and authentic—something worthy of their time and energy and in spite of all that tries to wear them down or block their way. Yet what I notice is that the first crucial step toward moving beyond limitations is not struggling against what is so but rather simply accepting the reality of the moment at hand.

To live fully, we need to accept all circumstances— joy and sadness, ease and uncertainty, and vibrant well-being as well as pain. It is best not to wait until times of crisis force us into thinking about learning acceptance. We can discover ways to really thrive rather than just survive by continually making the time to cultivate optimism, positive energy, trust, hope, and sense of connection. Only then can our choices become appropriately responsive, taking into consideration the very fullness of life.

There is an ancient story about a medieval monk who was asked how he practiced his faith within the confines and isolation of the monastery to which he had committed his life. His reply was, "I walk, I fall down, I get up." While it sounds simple, this is not so easy. And yet, isn't this exactly what is at the core of a life fully lived? None of us makes it through life unscathed. We make choices and take steps, and then we stumble or fall down. We make mistakes, and we become bruised and perhaps even battered along the way. Still, we pick ourselves up and do what needs to be done, step by wobbly step.

*there are days when
it would be all too easy
to slip into sadness
an ache here, a loss there
can be all too distracting
and depleting if we are not vigilant
in our heartful determination
to turn again and again
toward what might yet be
the gift in the grab bag
of what this moment has to offer*

there are times when
it would be oh so simple
to succumb to dismay
a disappointment here
a sudden recognition of
what never was or will be
can tearfully blind us from
finding some next more hopeful
or at least useful step

and so it is that
again and again
we must remind our whole self
of the preciousness of time
and the sweet possibilities
for love and kindness
for contribution and connection
that might be here still
waiting for us in the realms
of what we don't even know
we don't know

*d*on't get up
not so fast
don't just climb out of bed
not until you are good and ready
good spirited and ready minded
to greet the gift of this day

don't waste a move
struggling to untangle your
self from twisted sheets
and disturbing middle-night
meanderings of mind or spirit

stay still a moment longer
gather your wits and wonder
let kindness and hope
be the first blessings placed
carefully in your good and ready heart
as you begin to rise up

and welcome this new day
right here and now
spreading out before your eyes
inviting you onto a playground
of possibilities and into the unfolding
mystery of what it means
to be fully awake
and alive

Being with Sadness

How do we learn to be with sadness and not run from it? How do we plunge into the depths of our grief without losing ourselves there? Perhaps the key lies in not fighting against all that emotional energy but rather channeling it in some useful direction. In the course of a single life we must each confront so much sadness and loss as difficulties touch our lives and the lives of those we love. We have all known times when simply putting one foot in front of the other has seemed a monumental task in the face of great tragedy. And yet somehow we do it. By summoning our own inner strength and relying on the support of others, we can usually manage and make it through.

Mothers Against Drunk Driving (MADD) was started by Candace Lightner, a mother whose child was killed by someone driving irresponsibly while under the influence of alcohol. The concept of microlending was started by Muhammad Yunus, Harvard graduate and founder of the Grameen Bank, who was saddened by the great poverty he witnessed and motivated by his desire to do something to improve the lot of his own people in Bangladesh. Good people everywhere have done great things because they found a way to feel their sadness and use it rather than wallow in it.

Sometimes we use up the energy of our sadness dwelling on all that is wrong, unfair, bitter, or mean-spirited. We rant and rave until there is nothing left inside. Other times, we are able to hold our sadness more softly, allowing it to speak to us in its own voice without censure.

The blessing comes when, somewhere beyond the grieving and suffering, some little glimmer of light or lightness invites us to take a first small step. Beyond the drama and distress, we are shown some tiny thing that might be possible. Beyond the pity and the pain, we can be moved by something useful and good that has the capacity to enliven us once again.

There is a Sufi saying worth considering: "When the heart grieves over what it has lost, the spirit rejoices over what it has left." It takes great strength and courage to find some slight spark of gratitude deep within and allow for its warmth to spread through us. Yet it is the very kindling of that spark that allows us to make it through the dark and difficult times of our lives.

I walk this edge of sadness
and fear and insecurity
not wanting to fall in
balancing carefully on the rim
of a narrow wall of grief

precarious, that's how it feels as I
teeter from one emotion to another
blinded by the dark bias of loss upon loss
obscuring any vistas of possibility

in this place of weariness
hope seems a long way away
an exhausting distance to traverse
while I can barely muster the will and power
to simply do the next thing there is to do
but I do remember my ancient grandmother
forever uttering her simple prayer
"God, give me strength"

and so I, too, now
offer up these words of grace
to carry me through these tumultuous
and treacherous times
and curiously I am comforted
by the image of that wizened woman
placing her hands above me
and saying "a blessing on your head"

may it be so

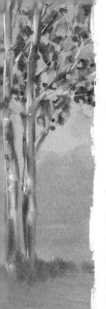

Forgiving and Letting Go

When we hold on to grievances and bitter stories about the past, there is a *cost* to us personally as well as to those we are unwilling to forgive. Carrying around so much anger and sadness can rob us of joy, energy, health, power, and a whole lot more. From that perspective, forgiveness becomes a courageous but necessary choice and a gift to oneself.

While we are usually aware and can be quite vocal about anger directed toward others, what is also true is that all too often our anger is self-directed. Each of us, it seems, has this nagging little inner critic who sits on our shoulder whispering nasty nothings into our ear about all the ways we are *less than* what we believe we should be. And, of course, there are all the ways that we have done things we wish we hadn't—wish we could undo, rewind the tape, or erase from the stories of our lives. Yet, as the Buddha said, "You, yourself, as much as anybody in the entire universe, deserve your love and affection." And, I would add, forgiveness.

Then, too, there is all the inner mind-chatter about the ways life has not turned out quite the way we, in our hopefulness, imagined it would. In the course of our lives, both choice and chance wreak havoc on all our wishful thinking and planning. And so, at some point in time and for the sake of our own inner peace, it becomes a question of forgiving ourselves the roads not taken in order to enjoy and celebrate the ones we have.

The Museum of Tolerance in Los Angeles has two entrances—one for tolerant people and the other for those who are intolerant. If you try to open the door of tolerance you will find that it is locked. Why? Because, of course, none of us is without bias or judgment. And therein lies another key to forgiveness. We each have opinions and prejudices, and it is only when we can recognize and forgive these that we can begin to make the shift to acceptance and forgiveness of others.

And so it is that there appear to be two sides to forgiveness. The first person we must bless with forgiveness is always ourself. Only then can we expand our openheartedness to another. Only then can we walk in the shoes of another and attempt to understand what prompted their words and/or actions. Only then can we embrace both our and their brokenness as an integral part of our common humanity.

how strong
my reluctance
to relinquish endless
inner lists of past failures
and inadequacies

how willing
my mind
to measure each
expectation and regret
by some harsh yardstick

how difficult
my resistance
to drop all preconceptions
born of "yes"
and "no"

how futile
my grasping
to hold on to what little I knew
for sure
just yesterday

how compelling
my longing
to experience at last
the simplicity
of unencumbered being

*t*o live fully
and well
we must befriend life
not as we wish it
to be but as it is
only by practicing
acceptance and
letting go
of endless expectations
and disappointments
can we greet each day
with arms and hearts
open wide enough
to beckon
into our embrace
the wholeness
of who we are and
all that might yet be
possible

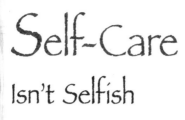

Self-Care
Isn't Selfish

Healing is a journey that happens in waves. Riding the peaks and valleys of those surges gracefully requires balance, focus, and a certain capacity to be fully present to each oncoming swell. The challenge is finding our own way to stay in the flow of it all, and that requires a loving commitment to ourselves.

We can be so generous when it comes to helping others. Yet all too often we fail to give ourselves that same measure of kindness and consideration. We put our needs on the back burner until things boil over and can no longer be ignored. Only then does the situation finally arouse our attention. But what if true and loving self-care were a way of life, rather than either an emergency measure or an afterthought? How might our attentiveness to ourselves before, during, and after whatever crisis befalls us change the course of events?

What does truly nurturing ourselves look like? It's not good enough to simply go through the motions of doing what we know we "should" do for ourselves. When approached with that mindset, we race through all these supposedly necessary "doings" without ever allowing ourselves to *be present* to the healing that is available in the midst of these activities.

And so, first of all, it is important to choose judiciously those healing and healthful practices that feed all aspects of ourselves. From good and nourishing foods to exercise that energizes and invigorates us, from pleasurable rituals to ample opportunities for quiet reflection, we each need to find our own authentic ways to honor ourselves by taking great care.

Consider the whole concept of MDRs. MDR is an acronym used to refer to the minimum daily requirements of essential nutrients that each body needs to function. Stretching that concept further and taking it to the next level, MDRs might also be the perfect way to refer to those *mindful daily restoratives and revitalizers* that allow us to feel truly well and nourished on all levels. They would include opportunities to eat well and nourish our bodies with adequate movement and exercise, while also allowing us time to replenish our spirit through play, laughter, and deep reflection. And, of course, we cannot ignore the need for ample rest. Remember that a full night's sleep each night really is one of the best healing gifts we can give ourselves. The possibilities for MDRs are all around us. We must choose thoughtfully and then make the commitment to devote time and attention to folding them into our lives each and every day. By doing so, we take long strides on the journey to our own healing and fullest capacity for enjoying life.

let today be a long, sweet drink
warm and satisfying as honeyed tea
allow yourself the easy pleasure
of even just a few unburdened
moments spent savoring
the simple joys of an intimate
exchange of words or touch
the special gift of an inspiring idea
or notion
found like a shiny penny
when and where you least expect it

let today be timeless
toss your watch into a drawer
and turn off for even just a little while
all the digital reminders
of each second ticking away
let the hours roll along instead
without notice or concern
while you allow yourself to be tossed
about gently on random waves
of thought or reverie
with neither purpose nor destination

allow yourself the simple luxury
of no thing and no where while
giving yourself permission
to settle into the rhythms and
counter-rhythms all around
playful riffs arising spontaneously
with no exacting plan of where
they are headed but rather a certain
unexpected delight by what shows up
in the spaciousness
of unfettered possibility

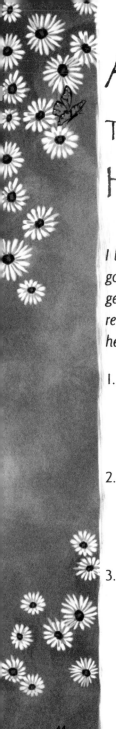

A Baker's Dozen of Things to Do on Your Healing Journey

I love the idea of a baker's dozen. It's about the extra goodie in the box that you are given as an act of generosity. Each special treat is an opportunity for replenishment that you can gift yourself with on your healing journey.

1. **Take a breath.** Take several—long, deep, full ones that expand your rib cage and nourish every cell with oxygen. Allow your breath to fill your soul and soothe your spirit.

2. **Stroll, walk, hike, bike, climb, run.** Move. And do so outside in the daylight for even just a little while because sunlight is a nutrient that is needed every day to stay healthy and alert.

3. **Move toward the merriment.** Joy is a magnet. Spend time with people who know how to stay upbeat and smiling, no matter what may be troubling them. While you are at it, follow Ralph Waldo Emerson's advice and "Sprinkle joy!" It's a potent weapon against everything from doldrums to despair.

4. **Take a long nap, a quick snooze, or a power pause.** Close your eyes. It may look like you're doing nothing, but on both the cellular and spiritual levels, you are using this time to repair and refresh your whole self.

5. *S t r e t c h.* Reach up and down and forward and back. Feel the blood flow and your body come alive.

6. **Take time out for a reality check.** Just how important is whatever you are momentarily crazed about anyway? Stop long enough to gain perspective and prioritize.

7. **Add color to your calendar.** Use colored pens to keep track of your daily activities. Think *pink* for pampering, *red* for exercise, *blue* for times with friends, and *purple* for the things that feed your spirit. The goal is to create *rainbow days*, but also remember to leave some white space for refreshing and revitalizing pauses.

8. **Take tea.** See how soothing and nurturing it feels. Become a tea connoisseur. A cup brewed to perfection is a tea-rific time-out.

9. **Create an intuition infusion.** Pause in the midst of the busyness of your day. Listen deeply to the steadfast voice within waiting to be heard above the clamor of all that vies for attention.

10. **Take a blessing break.** Name 'em, count 'em, and give thanks. You might want to keep a gratitude journal and make at least one entry daily. Notice how doing so makes you feel.

11. **Take a comfort check.** Scan your body and notice any little aches or areas of tightness, and give them some loving touch and attention.

12. **Cultivate your inner smile.** Think of something silly that amuses you, and allow a smile to form at the edges of your mouth. Let that smile turn into tinglings of happiness that spread inwardly like a special secret. Imagine that inner smile traveling all through you, making the rounds to each and every cell and leaving your insides radiant with joy. Visualize that smile becoming more and more difficult to contain until it finally bursts into a great big grin that lights up your face and spreads contagiously to everyone in your presence.

13. **Feel the wonder.** Make time to notice the small and great wonders all around you. There are so many ways to quite simply be reverent and in awe of life.

Moving Past Fear

Perhaps distress over the unknown or what's ahead is holding you in the grip of fear. We have each known that feeling of being frozen—unable to navigate even just one next step, let alone a possible future beyond the current catastrophic moment. But later, after surviving that point in time, we can look back with a new and expanded view and see not just the challenges but also the possibilities seeded in them.

There must be something deeply human about this capacity. Again and again, we hear stories of those who lost their jobs, their homes, their health, or a loved one, yet they were somehow slowly, often painfully, able to move beyond their fearful situation to arrive at a place they could not have imagined for themselves.

Do you ever wish you could say to a loved one, "Don't be so afraid. Hang in there. Trust me. I've been there, and life, love, and laughter may still lie waiting beyond the bend." Yet words can feel so inadequate or even dangerously insensitive, no matter our good intentions and worldly experience. Why is it that we must each discover all this for ourselves? Perhaps it is because by doing so, we just might be transformed in the process.

One thing that can help us to face our fear when it rears its ugly head is the FEAR acronym—Flimsy Evidence (or False Expectations) Appearing Real. When we can remember to take a careful look at what we are reacting to so seriously, we can sometimes discern what is actually happening. Generally, we will find there is some element of our own "awfulizing" or "catastrophizing" involved and that, mostly, it is the unknown that has us in a tailspin. When we take a few deep breaths to become more centered, we can begin to quiet our palpitating heart. From this calmer perspective, we can start to ponder what the interFEARence is and how we might best respond rather than just react.

how easily my stomach can
tie itself up in "nots"
tangled up with fears of scarcity
and a doom and gloom sense
of impotence and insufficiency
in the face of who knows what
lies ahead

failing to make time to fully take in
what is not only so
but also what might yet be possible
I plunge instead into the muck
of half-truths and helplessness

it all feels so familiar
this inner turmoil that coils round
and round itself like a cat
chasing its tail and kicking up
dust in its frantic wake
but what I also know
is that perspectives can shift
and change as quickly as the light
and shadow now playing on the
walls of my discontent...

what I also know is that grace
can arrive on the wings of a kind
word or a strong hand or
an encouraging thought that
drifts toward me from a lectern
or book or on the waves
of my own sweet dreams

and so in the absence of courage
or a clear sense of how to move
beyond knee-jerk reactivity
to thoughtful responsiveness
what experience has shown me
is to allow faith and patience
to find their way to me
curled up here in my corner of concern
and to comfort me
for however long it takes to get
my bearings and summon the
wherewithal and understanding
to simply move on

Getting Unstuck

All living creatures get stuck sometimes. It seems none of us are exempt. But unlike our furry friends and crawling creatures, it's not always being physically stuck that keeps us wedged in or pulled down. More often than not, there's a logjam of emotions and limiting beliefs that holds us back from going with the flow of life. Whenever we are struggling to heal from something, we must begin by feeling our way through whatever is keeping us from getting into action.

The good news is that, sooner or later, we are often graced with an easing of constrictions as the scale tips toward our capacity for love, hope, and resilience. And so it seems that what we need to do in times of confinement and confusion is just keep breathing and keep looking for wiggle room.

breathe in
expand and receive life

breathe out
let that which no longer serves you fall away...

breathe in
allow grace to enter your heart

breathe out
usher out all that would sully your holy space

breathe in
be inspired by miracles all around you

breathe out
gently exhale mundane concerns

breathe in
invite the gift of life's creative force into each cell

breathe out
release spent energy and in exchange

breathe in
the refreshing newness and possibility of just
this moment

breathe out
fears, fatigue, frustrations that weigh you down

breathe in
and let life fill you with joy

breathe out
offer the precious gift of yourself to the world

When it happens
when we come unstuck
how serendipitous it all seems
as the missing pieces fall into place
and puzzling pictures
become vistas of opportunity

when the logjam finally releases
when things at last start to flow
how marvelous it all becomes
as our accumulated biases and limiting beliefs
are washed away
by a stream of newfound hope

when the hard knot in our belly eases
when our lungs open to receive a full breath of life
how refreshing it all feels
as the confinements and constrictions
of our small fears crumble
in the face of our expanding capacity
for love and joy

when it happens
when the heart and mind open
how miraculous it all appears to be
as the detritus and dramas
of our small worldview disappear
in the wake of our willingness
to embrace the adventure
of being fully alive

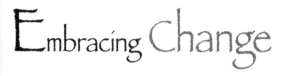

Embracing Change

The nature of life is impermanence and change. What causes us to suffer and drains our energy is simply our refusal to accept this fact. At the extreme ends of a long continuum of how we as humans deal with change are two diametrically opposed strategies. The first one is grounded in our great fear of the unknown—of being out of control; so we sometimes try to cling with all our might to the status quo—the safe and familiar. The other strategy is to simply let go and *go with the flow* of life. While each approach involves using our "energy," clinging requires the greater expenditure. It can be frustrating and fruitless, stressful and exhausting. On the other hand, allowing ourselves to be carried by life's flow can leave us refreshed and renewed.

Being able to shift into a positive mindset when faced with life's uncertainties can help generate a feeling of vital aliveness because it allows us to remain open to surprise, wonder, and possibility. To *be in the flow* means to be totally present to what's going on around us while simultaneously focusing and directing our energy in the direction of our intentions and commitments.

Staying in the flow is a lifelong process. Our task is to surf the waves that come our way while staying awake and aware, balanced and centered, ready and open to the manner in which life unfolds. There are many ways we can allow change to energize us by preparing for and managing our response to the inevitable shifts and oscillations that life brings. Here are a few:

1. Embrace change as the very sum and substance of life. Find ways to welcome, with a sense of anticipation rather than dread, the endless stream of new challenges and chances that are constantly arising.

2. A strong and resilient body is the best foundation for supporting change. Be committed to your own extraordinary self-care by taking time to eat properly, get adequate rest (including wonderful rejuvenating naps and meditative moments), and exercise to build strength and stamina.

3. Cultivate a resilience of mind. Become a lifelong learner, continually in the process of exploration and discovery as a way to "grow" with the flow and participate fully in life.

4. Living successfully is about making wise choices again and again. As things change—and they will—engage in an ongoing, soul-searching inquiry about what you are passionate about saying "Yes!" to and what you choose to say "No!" to... NOW in this moment. Focus on what really matters and brings you great joy, and don't be reluctant to let go of that which no longer serves or energizes you.

5. Practice being present in each moment. No matter the turbulence of life, there is always a still, center point of peacefulness. Meditation, journal writing, prayer, simple rituals, yoga, and deep, focused breathing are all ways to access a sense of focused presence.

6. Learn to laugh at life's calamities rather than bemoan and groan about them. The good news is that beyond allowing us to lighten up and cope more readily, laughter is good for us. Studies show that when we laugh, our blood pressure falls, circulation increases, pain decreases, delivery of oxygen and nutrients to tissues improves, breathing capacity expands, and our immune system becomes heartier and more active against viruses and cancer. Wow! And there's more. Laughter diminishes the secretion of stress hormones, like cortisol and epinephrine, making it the perfect natural stress reliever.

No matter our well-laid plans, life continues to unfold in unforeseen and mysterious ways. Rather than resisting change, may your life be blessed with the magic and mystery of it all.

Oh, blue sky of
living, breathing joy
and here I am
still a witness
to broad brushstrokes of
impossibly white clouds
highlighted by a late
afternoon golden lining
of luminosity and
dare I say hope?

turning the corner
how can I take in
the covenant of color
that stretches across
my very own
road to the very place
I call home
gracing my entry into
however many years may yet
stretch before me?

how is it that the world
seems so much more
exquisite just when
we have come through a dark
tunnel of wondering whether
we might be expunged
or expelled from the grace
of still belonging here?...

and how pray tell
shall I live my
days in the wake
of receding fear
and grief?

how many ways
are there to write
with broad brushstrokes
of gratitude across
the canvas of the
coming years?
how many covenants
of colorful, joyful
love-filled words
can I spread across
the hours of the days
that stretch before me
each one a brand-new
golden promise
of possibility?

Invite Magic into Your Life

We've been taught from early childhood the value of having a realistic plan and specific goals, which can also be interpreted as the importance of not leaving too much to chance. We have also been educated to believe that miracles are little more than a fool's wishfulness or wishful foolishness. And yet, there are everyday miracles happening all around us. As David Ben-Gurion is often quoted as saying, "Anyone who doesn't believe in miracles isn't a realist."

More recently, as we have gained awareness about the power of our thoughts to impact our physical reality, we have even been encouraged to tap into this capability by visualizing precise outcomes and positively affirming their manifestation. *Ahhhh, but...* the trick is to leave room for the unexpected and unanticipated. Positive affirmations and creative, uplifting visualizations are awesome techniques to add positive energy to our dreams, as long as we remain open to something beyond our best imaginings happening. The most effective way I know to do this is to always include the prayerful phrase, "May either this or something better manifest." The limitless options that the universe may have in store for us are oftentimes beyond our ability to picture in our mind's eye. By keeping the door open, we invite magic in.

So how do you begin to allow for more magic in your life? Here are four possible steps to consider.

1. **Define Magic.** Understand that magic isn't about rabbits coming out of hats—that's simply illusion. Anytime a wonderful coincidence happens that is beyond the realm of your expectations or directed efforts, it just might be an affirmation that magic is in the air.

2. **Expect Magic.** You can take a realistic approach to life's everyday events and still believe in magical possibilities... things that happen that defy simple logic.

3. **Recognize Magic.** When magic happens, don't ignore or reject it because it's not part of your plan or preconceived notion. Whenever something serendipitous or unexpected comes your way, open yourself up to new opportunities. Tap into your intuitive inklings and knowings in order to recognize that something special or out of the ordinary is happening.

4. **Celebrate Magic.** Take time to acknowledge the small moments of sweet reprieves and simple pleasures that may be tucked in between the more challenging times. Whenever possible, bring to your life an attitude of gratitude. By recognizing and giving thanks for your blessings, you invite more in.

forget for a moment
how you came to be
here or why
and simply
be

leave aside all
the cumbersome maps
which are after all
mere measurements that
cannot fathom or touch
the holy ground
on which you now stand

yes, you have journeyed far
but are your eyes open wide enough
with wonder to take in
this mysterious moment
at the crossroads of here and now?

because there is, of course
no turning back
all those yesterdays
are but blessed bends
along the road to today
where now is always
a beginning

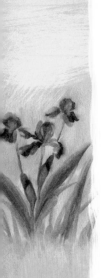

Easy Matters

When times are dark and difficult, we often find ourselves struggling with what's so. And yet at these crucial times, it is more important than ever to ease up and give oneself a chance to replenish and recover. In an ideal stress-less world, there is a certain rhythm of alternating between productively doing and simply being. In the midst of a crisis, the question becomes less about what you are doing and more about how you are being.

To begin to answer that question, it helps to simply notice where your attention and your energy are being directed. Are you buying into how hard life is? Are you attending to the day and its tasks, focusing on your never-ending to-do list with dread or a sense of drudgery? Or are you able to find, somewhere in the midst of it all, a sense of ease?

It seems that nowadays people worry more than ever. So much concern about the economy, the environment, and everything else has caused an apparent stress overload. The burdensome sense of "it is all too much" has cast a shadow across our capacity for ease and levity. But what both common sense and science tell us is that too much stress without regular reprieves is harmful to our health, our sense of happiness, and our ability to be creative and productive.

Sometimes we just need to "get easy," and we can begin by developing an *easy mind*. There is an interesting exercise that involves finding ways to reframe our thoughts in order to reclaim our best self and our best life. Draw a line down the middle of a piece of paper. On the left side, make a list of all the concerns, challenges, and supposedly negative events in your life right now. On the opposite side, do some reframing to shift your perspective by finding a blessing or positive possibility in each item. For example, if money is an issue, what are creative and perhaps even amusing ways you can spend less? Consider everything from an inexpensive family cook-in to expanding your wardrobe by swapping clothes with friends. Got a health issue? Could the blessing be that as you seriously make the time to take great care, you might just wind up healthier and in better shape?

Another way to shift your frame of mind is to change from "have to" to "get to." This revelation came to me from an older friend who showed up at exercise class one day and explained that she almost didn't come because she was in an "I have to go to yoga" frame of mind. Then she realized with a flash of gratitude that at her age, it is a great blessing to get to go to yoga. From a certain vantage point, we "get to do" a lot of things; for example, the laundry (which means we have clothes to wash and often a machine to wash them in) and the dishes (which means that there was food on our table and water in our faucet). We get to clean our homes and go to work and even pay taxes because we are fortunate enough for that to be possible.

Next, how about expanding your *easy heart?* Is there any anger lurking around in the dark corners of your mind that might be constricting your heartfulness? Try shining a light on those negative feelings, and find one thing you can do now to begin to sweep them away. Perhaps it is time to have a healing conversation with someone or to write a never-to-be-sent letter to put the negativity to rest. What about resentments? We all harbor regrets and perhaps even annoyances about roads not traveled— the woulda, coulda, shouldas of life. What would it take to forgive yourself by focusing instead on appreciating the choices that have made you who you are today?

Finally, give yourself a break by learning to have *easy eyes*. Instead of scrutinizing every flaw, soften your gaze to take in the larger picture. Health and wholeness are not about perfection. Rather what matters is being able to embrace all aspects of ourselves as integral parts of our lives. When we learn to give up on perfection and practice loving our whole self, we give ourself permission to blossom like flowers that miraculously arise through the cracks and imperfections in the sidewalk.

finding joy

Sometimes my joy is right there
on the pillow next to me
waiting for me to wake up
to wrap myself in its crimson cloak
and to dance into my day
bright-eyed and easy
other times I must reach out
way beyond my comfort zone
to grab and lay claim
to the happiness that is mine to choose
if I will but focus and do what it takes
to seize my day

sometimes there seems to be enough
pain in the world
to swallow me whole
and deposit me bleary-eyed and bone tired
in the belly of the whale and yet
it is that same wholeness
that delivers the key to my release

other times something as simple as sunshine
or the loyalty of a friend shining through for me
or the sweetness of a special kiss
or a lover's touch
can be enough to open my eyes
to a certain lightness of being
that is mine for the taking

wishing you
everyday miracles

*W*hen all heaven breaks loose
and you are showered
with the simple blessing
of a sunshiny moment
can you, will you stop
whatever has you in a muddle
and let gratitude spread out
all around you?

meandering through a field
of fragrant dreams and brilliantly
wild-flowering ideas popping up
here and there
can you, will you break
away from whatever has you so
tied up in "nots" and simply allow
possibility to take root
and blossom?

when you find yourself lost
in a forest of all that never was
or will be
can you, will you abandon
your useless maps and
let yourself navigate
by your own true heart
with a mind set for miracles?

perhaps if you are willing
and wise or just tired
of the old ways
and the limitations
of your old worldview
you can and you will
climb at last onto higher ground
and enjoy the panorama
and grandeur of life
in all its complex magnificence

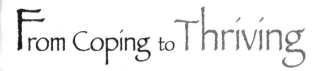

From Coping to Thriving

Coping is about getting by, making do, hanging in, and hanging on. It is a hand-to-mouth way of enduring and a necessary skill that we as humans have learned and perfected over thousands of years. We could not have survived otherwise.

But as humans, we are also driven to move beyond surviving to thriving, which is a far more engaging and enlivening way of being. In order to move past the drudgery of coping and add immeasurable richness to our lives, we must seek and cultivate the spark of hope that we carry within us. Often that hope lies outside the realm of what we know (or think we know). Since life is all about flow and flux and everything depends on everything else, sometimes we must simply wait in the quiet of the unknown and listen with all our heart. When we move beyond our constant struggle to bring logic and legitimacy to every situation, other feasibilities and ways of knowing, being, and doing begin to reveal themselves. The essential practice is to listen well rather than prematurely stifle or dissipate what is beginning to gather at the edges of our long-held opinions and judgments.

To live fully, we need to accept the whole gamut of circumstances in which we find ourselves as well as all the feelings those experiences engender—joy and sadness, ease and uncertainty, vibrant well-being and pain. We can only discover ways to truly thrive rather than just survive by continually cultivating optimism, positive energy, trust, hope, and a sense of connection. It's not just about rebounding in times of crisis, but also about maintaining joy in our daily lives.

The Spanish word for sunflower is *girasol*, which means turning toward the sun. Perhaps we can take a lesson from nature and learn to continually turn toward the sun—no matter the clouds and storms that temporarily block our access—as a way to re-source our energy and be replenished in the process.

Wake up, wake up
to the glorious glow of
this shiny, new day

have you gone to sleep
in the woods of hopelessness?
if so, step outside
your saga of sadness

dress yourself
in the glad rags of gratitude
and open wide your heart of hearts
to welcome in new visitors bearing
tidings of comfort and joy

embrace gifts of forgiveness
and merciful understanding
all wrapped up with a bow of
encouragement

the sun is bursting
with bright possibilities
shining lavishly wherever there is
a welcoming crack or opening

and all there is for you to do
is to loosen your grip on the past
and gratefully accept this present
shiny, new moment

True Acceptance

God, grant me the serenity to accept the people I cannot change, the courage to change the one I can, and the wisdom to know that person is me.

— *Someone Wise*

What does it mean to be accepting? *Webster's Dictionary* offers lots of definitions, but the key ideas are "to receive willingly" and to "endure without protest or reaction." It is to be at peace with whatever is happening. The question becomes, how do we arrive at that mindset? Certainly true acceptance lies way beyond both the things and situations we must come to terms with in the course of even a single day.

I read once that in the midst of a terrible drought, Navajo Indians do not pray for rain. Rather they create a ceremony to restore themselves to a state of harmony with the lack of water and with the dying crops and sheep all around them. Their practice is designed to allow for recognition of what is beyond human power to alter and to encourage a change of attitude that allows them to be at peace with the current reality.

This does not imply inaction or complacency. It is not about giving up and failing to go in search of water. It is not about being irresponsible with conserving and rationing what water there is. It is about being able to remain at peace in the midst of whatever is going on and whatever needs to be done. There are times when we make the decision to be content with what is so. Yet other times, there is a contented feeling of acceptance that simply washes over us, delivering us to some easy inner spaciousness we might not have come to by our own will alone.

There are four rather concise rules of life that I have heard repeated time and again: First, show up. Next, pay attention. Third, tell the truth. Fourth, don't be attached to the outcome. It seems that when we can show up fully, when we can pay attention to what has both meaning and heart, when we can speak our truth with neither judgment nor blame, and when we can allow ourselves to be open to opportunities without being attached to specific outcomes, we can begin to ease into that place of true acceptance. What is astonishing is that it's when we are most in alignment with what is so that we are least aware of it. We must learn to live and breathe within the spaciousness of peace and joy. Only when these are absent do we become cognizant of what is missing. Perhaps, during these times, what we need most is a fine-tuning of our awareness.

*W*hat might you be willing
to let stay
unresolved
incomplete, unfixed?

what burden could you
lay down by the side
of the road and then
without ever looking back
continue on your way?

what last straw would you
leave unturned and unexamined
in order to lighten your load
enough to soar on the winds
of something as simple
and satisfying as
unimpeded joy?

what might you allow
to go unlisted
undated, undone
so as to release the tethers
holding you fixed
and anchored to obligations
that have chosen
and been chosen by
you?...

what could you relinquish and
what price would you gladly pay
for the precious privilege
of quiet contentment
and could you
without regrets
leave furled the flag
of endless achievements
in order to surrender to
the holy sweetness of
unencumbered being?

life is feeling softer now
as I learn to abandon big plans
and long-term goals complete
with all sorts of fancy strategic plots
and simply settle into
the next right thing

life is tasting sweeter now
as I learn to delight in
just that morsel of pleasure
just this fragrant morning
gifted to me as inexplicably
as life itself

beyond the exhaustion of
endless striving and perpetual
walls to scale
there is this other way
that is becoming
available to the extent
that I can loosen the yoke of
insufficiency
to which I have for so long
hitched myself...

it has taken the turmoil of years
and the considerable sweat equity
of endlessly trying so very hard
to do what I insist
must be done
yet now the simple truth
that less might truly be more
has taken me by surprise
as I can at last
surrender into the satisfaction
of a day well lived

finally
as feelings of overwhelm fall away
I am finding myself satisfied
by the easy presence of just here
just now and just this
next right thing
more and more at peace
with whatever life brings
because it is quite simply
what is so

Something Larger Is at Play

Do you sometimes find yourself worrying about all that is not going according to your plan and all that is not bending to your worldview of how things should be? No matter how carefully and creatively we design our days and, by extension, our lives, LIFE happens.

During times like these, have you ever had the feeling that something larger is at play and you are being mysteriously guided in ways that are somehow aligned with your soul's great yearnings? When you pay attention and can see the fuller picture, perhaps your response can blessedly shift to one of gratitude.

There are gratitude moments around us all the time if we remember to look. One of the most valuable exercises we can do to increase our capacity for health and happiness is to take time to pay attention and perhaps to even write down things for which we are grateful. Keeping a "gratitude journal" can be a powerful tool to remind us to bask in the blessings of our life, to expand our sense of hope, and to strengthen our capacity for healing.

Sometimes I sit in wasteful worry
agitated by all that refuses to bend
to my will or wishfulness
while there on the wall
the cuckoo sounds out timely reminders
of the craziness of my small worldview

sometimes I stare unseeing
into the vast spaciousness of my unlived days
unable to muster momentum or passion
yet there on my shelf are volumes
of eloquent words of wisdom and wonder
reminding me of other realities
waiting to be lived

sometimes I wallow in futile
whimperings and regrets
stuck in bygones about all
that never was or will ever be
yet here in this moment
my heart is beating steadily onward
and my mind is steadfastly aware
that there is more, so much more
than meets my small "I"
it is then that my deeper self
remembers the goodness of my days and
recalling one by one the blessings of this life
can recognize and open to
blessings yet to come

I give thanks because I must
because my soul sings with such
great fullness
because the butterflies are
so beautiful
so symmetrical and so I must
stop in a chapel and give thanks
prayerfully, reverently
without knowing to whom
exactly or how

because life is so grand and so difficult
because blessings arrive unbidden
because prayers are answered or not
and yet life flows on
with gifts beyond our meager
imaginings and hopes
brought to us by some grand design or not
it does not matter

I offer thoughts of gratitude because I must
because the only responsible
response to the beauty of
a bird in flight or
the harshness of the winter's
storm is awe and
because I am struck speechless
by the tenderness of the male
cardinal feeding the female...

that I have lived to see
such things
that I have survived and
thrived for all these years
that I have made it through
fears and tears and
night sweats and sweet dreams
and mornings of such magnificence
is quite simply miraculous
and so I am left breathless
struck dumb and delighted
by all that we mere humans
inadequately call life

I give thanks because
in my heart of hearts
I believe or
simply want to believe
that there is some unnamable
force in this dazzling universe
that receives my thankfulness
that understands my awe
that welcomes my prayerful
ponderings and praises
and that holds me
and all that lives
in an embrace of everlasting love

It Takes as Long as It Takes

Remember when you were a child sitting in the back seat of the car and driving your parents crazy by asking, "Are we there yet?" When we are in the thick of a healing journey, that same impatience to be "there" already can haunt us, leaving us feeling both restless and disappointed rather than able to enjoy what is all around us waiting to be experienced along the way.

The truth is that ultimately there really isn't any "there" to get to. Rather there is an ongoing series of now moments that become available to us when we are prepared to simply notice what is happening in any particular segment of time. It is also important to recognize that healing is not necessarily the same as finding a "cure" or having things be exactly the way they were before. When we can just attend to our wounds, doing our best to seek ways to heal and feel more at ease in each moment, we come to realize that this simple act can be a source of exquisite comfort and peace.

Learning to love and care for ourselves requires, above all, a willingness to trust in the process of being fully present and open to life. This can

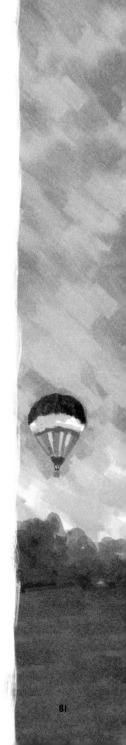

include seeking inspiration in nature, in prayer, in rituals, and in the words and expertise of others, as well as relying on our own intuitive inklings and moment-by-moment experiences.

While we might want to rush through the tough stuff so we can get to the place where everything is finally okay, it's probably neither sensible nor particularly healing to do so. By choosing to live in the thinnest slice of time we can define for ourselves, we allow things to unfold rather than unravel in the wake of our frenetic attempts to merely patch things up.

There is much to be learned along the way. Chances are, if we pay attention to the small shifts and changes, we will be able to find both joy and hope on our journey. If we do not repel the difficulties we encounter or try too hard to cling only to the best moments, the lack of struggle will bring with it the gifts of peace and perhaps unexpected new opportunities.

Sometimes
it all depends
on that fraction of time when
I remember to stop
long enough
for my soul to catch up

sometimes
everything hinges
on that moment in time when
I am asked to yield the floor because
through that necessary pause
I come to recognize the gift
embedded in being moved aside
long enough for my soul
to glimpse another way

sometimes
as life teeters on the edge
of that point in time when
I am so tangled in a web
of my own making that
there seems to be no way out
grabbing hold
requires finding the still point
where my soul can intuit its way
through the whole messy maze...

sometimes
as I thrash around in the deep waters
of my bizarre busyness
I finally realize that
only by surrendering into the dark stillness
can my soul at last rise to the surface
buoyed by the sweet
currents of my most authentic self

Consider the Miracle
of a Seed

Have you ever actually witnessed the miracle of a seed growing into the food that sustains life? Miraculously lush offerings can come from one simple seed.

Now consider how a small seed of hope or a tiny inkling of possibility or a mere glimmer of a new idea can, if carefully planted and gently tended, grow into an amazing lushness that takes hold as a brand-new reality.

Perhaps you feel as if you are standing alone in a barren wasteland where dreams have been plowed under and old prospects and expectations have turned into a tangle of weeds.

Please don't lose heart. Even life's saddest moments can turn into fertile ground for something new to take root and push small green shoots up toward the ever waiting light of day. What are the seeds you yearn to plant? Now is the time and wherever you are is the place. Just begin.

When the world beats
all too heavily at the door
how can we hold on to
the wonder of being alive?

when sorrow comes flooding
over the dam of our best
efforts to keep disaster at bay
how can we still grasp
the amazement of being alive?

what has become
abundantly clear
after years of being bowled over
and swept under
is simply this

the miracle of a beating heart
or the beating wings of a dragonfly
or the winged wildness of a bird in flight
or the wild beauty of a stormy night
or the beautiful magic of a seed
taking root
can all tilt the scale
toward awe
if we can simply turn our attention
toward the astonishing magnitude
and magnificence of this
and every moment.

rainbows

there are always
rainbows waiting beyond
even the most turbulent storms
bridges of hope extending
their invitation to seek
the next pot of golden possibilities

and always the sun waits
patiently shining
beyond even the most
oppressive bleakness
and like a sunflower
I have only to turn
in the direction of the light
for the shadows to fall away
behind me

when life throws a curve ball or
a crushing blow to the gut
and I'm down for the count
wind and will knocked out of me
thrown off course
disoriented and in disarray
with no clear compass to steer by
no breeze to fill my soul...

still even in the stillness
I must remember that
the wind is there
stirring somewhere over the
rainbow gaining force
and true north remains
true no matter how
the moment obscures
my bearings

soon, very soon
I will, I pray, right myself
and find my right course
grab hold of my rudder
and sail on in the direction
of my true calling

and for now
simply holding on to hope
gives me the courage
to carry on

Hope Is a Choice

There are thousands of things that can give us hope and just as many things that can take it away. Babies give me hope. Good teachers, good parents, and good citizenship give me hope, as well as the willingness to be in an ongoing discourse about what all that means. Good music, art, literature, and beautifully crafted objects give me hope about our infinite creative capacity. Simple acts of kindness and generosity give me hope as do stories of commitment and dedication to anything meaningful and worthwhile. Technology gives me hope. There are breakthroughs happening in medicine and alternative energy resources that may one day save our bodies from the worst ravages of disease and our planet from the more destructive activities of humankind.

What is clear is that hope needs to be a choice we make again and again. I am aware that the half-full glass only appears to be so when I am disposed to declare it so and live as if it is so. And I am also certain that when I choose hope and lean toward optimism, possibility, and recovery, the great blessing is that healing happens on many levels and happiness shows up in my life in many ways.

What is hope anyway
a certain ease with uncertainty
a certain inclination toward possibility
and anticipation of serendipity
it is the disappearing art
of patient attentiveness
to things and non-things
that shimmer in the distance

star wishers
and penny-in-the-well tossers
know about hope
as do children
gazing in store windows
and pioneers blazing new trails
through the wilderness

hope dances and skips and runs circles
around stodgy skeptics
ruminating on doom and gloom
for only those who can
cozy up to dreams while tackling life
with goodwill and willingness
can truly appreciate
the miracles waiting to be born
of an idea shaped
by language and love
by belief and the abandonment of resistance
into exquisite form

there comes a time
when the real healing begins
beyond the myriad interventions
and miracles of medicine
beyond the mysterious ways of
herbal decoctions and nutritious concoctions
beyond the magic of touch
and graceful movements mindfully practiced
something shifts somehow
and we know deep in our bones
that we have been reborn into
our own magnificent wholeness

steeped in gratitude
for all that has sustained us
and carried us along
to this blessed moment
we experience at last
the vital essence of our aliveness
and the responsiveness of our mind and body
to the love that is always there
at the very core of our being
and at the very edges of
our own glorious wholeness

and so at last we bask in the fullness
of this precious journey called life
and the expansiveness of
our own timeless spirit

Thank you, dear reader, for spending time meandering through all that I have gathered here. My hope is that these words have somehow touched your spirit, comforted your mind, inspired your fortitude, and eased your way along your healing journey.

Take great care,

— Minx Boren